111 Dumbbell Workouts

Book for Men and Women

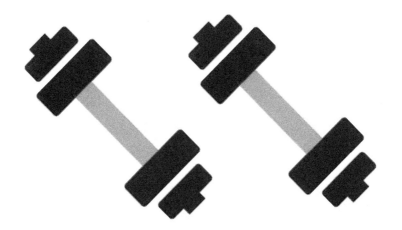

111 Dumbbell Workouts
Book for Men and Women

111 Workouts to
Build Muscle and Lose Fat

> Extra Logging Sheets & Videos to Watch Exercises
> <u>Are Available by Scanning QR Codes</u>

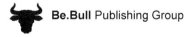

Be.Bull Publishing Group

Toronto, Canada

The original purchaser of this book has permission to reproduce the pages of this book for personal use only. No other parts of this publication may be reproduced in whole or in part, shared with others, stored in a retrieval system, digitized, or transmitted in any form without written permission from the publisher.

Copyright 2021, Be.Bull Publishing Group (Aria Capri International Inc). All rights reserved.

Authors:

Be.Bull Publishing Group

Devon Abbruzzese & Mauricio Vasquez

First Printing: July 2022

ISBN- 978-1-990709-51-7

FREE DOWNLOAD

BONUS No 1

ALL LOGGING SHEETS from this book are available *FOR NO EXTRA COST* for you by scanning a QR code.

You can scan the QR code, print, and record your workouts to measure your performance as many times as you want.

(The QR is found at the end of this book)

BONUS No 2 -

VIDEOS for ALL EXERCISES ARE AVAILABLE to check how the exercises are to be performed

(The QR codes are found at the end of this book)

Unlock Your Fitness Potential with Artificial Intelligence

I am thrilled to introduce a groundbreaking tool, *"AI-Powered Training Coach" GPT*, for physical fitness, developed with the latest advancements in AI technology. This advanced tool is designed to enhance your workout experience, offering personalized exercise plans tailored to your preferences, needs, and the equipment you have available.

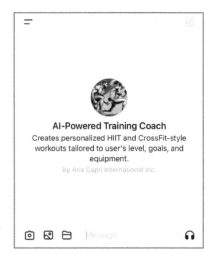

AI-Powered Training Coach
Creates personalized HIIT and CrossFit-style workouts tailored to user's level, goals, and equipment.
By Aria Capri International Inc.

This innovative AI system, utilizing Generative Pre-trained Transformer (GPT) technology by OpenAI.com, is specifically programmed to support your fitness journey. It acts as a dynamic fitness companion, aligning with your personal fitness goals and the resources at your disposal, providing custom-tailored workout routines and fitness advice.

Engaging with this AI tool is incredibly user-friendly and intuitive. Upon access, you'll be presented with a straightforward interface where you can input your fitness objectives, available equipment, and other relevant details. The AI processes this information rapidly, delivering tailored workout plans and suggestions almost instantly.

Whether your goal is to build muscle, increase endurance, or simply maintain a healthy lifestyle, this AI tool is your gateway to a more effective and personalized fitness experience.

Included in this section there are a couple of screenshots displaying the user interface you'll encounter when accessing this unique fitness AI tool. This visual guide offers a clear overview of the tool's functionality, assisting you in your first steps towards a smarter, AI-enhanced workout regimen.

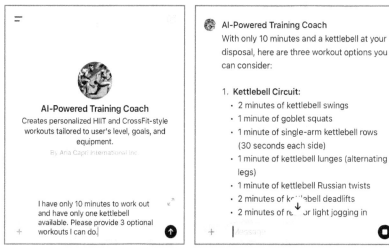

To embark on your journey towards achieving your fitness goals with the support of this innovative AI technology, please go to this link
https://mindscapeartwork.ck.page/trainingcoachgpt
or scan this QR code.

Go to the link or scan the QR code shown below to check out other workout books

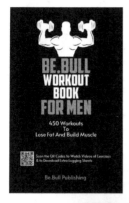 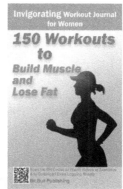 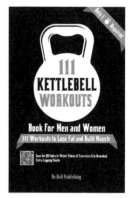

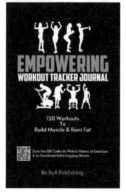 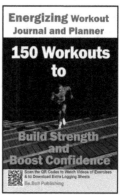

https://linktr.ee/be.bull

<u>TIPS</u>

- Adjust the weight of the dumbbells, the number of repetitions and the time cap for the workouts according to your capabilities, skills and physical condition
- Listen to your body and don't push yourself too hard
- If you don't have enough space where to run, you can do jumping jacks. 100-meter run is approximately equivalent to 50 jumping jacks
- Walk into the gym with a workout already selected for you
- Get motivated with a fun workout playlist
- Put your phone on airplane mode
- Start your workout with some stretches
- Pick the right weight - you will notice that the workouts don't indicate a specific weight. That is on purpose. Just choose a weight that is right for you.
- Log the details of each workout so you can track your progress. You can track the weight, time and number of repetitions
- Enjoy your workouts

Disclaimer

1. Be.Bull Publishing (Aria Capri International Inc.) strongly recommends that you consult with your physician before beginning any exercise program or workout. You should be in good physical condition and be able to participate in the exercises and workouts. We are not a licensed medical care provider and represents that we have no expertise in diagnosing, examining, or treating medical conditions of any kind, or in determining the effect of any specific exercise or workout on a medical condition.

2. You should understand that when participating in any exercise or workout, there is the possibility of physical injury. If you engage in the exercises and workouts of this book, you agree that you do so at your own risk, are voluntarily participating in these activities, assume all risk of injury to yourself, and agree to release and discharge Be.Bull Publishing (Aria Capri International Inc.) from any and all claims or causes of action, known or unknown, arising out of this book and videos.

3. The information provided through this book is not intended to be a substitute for professional medical advice, diagnosis or treatment. Never disregard professional medical advice, or delay in seeking it, because of something you have read on this book or watch in the videos. Never rely on information on this book or videos in place of seeking professional medical advice.

4. Be.Bull Publishing (Aria Capri International Inc.) is not responsible or liable for any advice, course of treatment, diagnosis or any other information, services or products that you obtain through this book or videos. You are encouraged to consult with your doctor with regard to the information contained on or through this book or videos. After reading this book or watching videos from this book, you are encouraged to review the information carefully with your professional healthcare provider.

WORKOUTS	Day 1 Reps / Time / Weight	Day 2 Reps / Time / Weight	Day 3 Reps / Time / Weight	Day 4 Reps / Time / Weight	Day 5 Reps / Time / Weight
1 12 Rounds for Time of: •6 Dumbbell Push-Ups •12 Dumbbell Hang Squat Cleans					
2 •10 Dumbbell man-makers (Split reps between arms) •12 Burpees •500-meter Run •36 Air Squats •12 Hand-release push-ups					
3 10 Rounds for Time of: •250 meter Run •15 Deadlift Burpee Dumbbells					
4 3 Rounds for Time of: •1,000-meter Run •30 Dumbbell Squat Cleans					
5 10 Rounds for Time of: •10 Dumbbell man-makers (Split reps between arms) •20 Dumbbell Deadlifts					

WORKOUTS		Day 6	Day 7	Day 8	Day 9	Day 10
		Reps / Time / Weight	Reps / Time / Weight	Reps / Time / Weight	Reps / Time / Weight	Reps / Time / Weight
1	12 Rounds for Time of: •6 Dumbbell Push-Ups •12 Dumbbell Hang Squat Cleans					
2	•10 Dumbbell man-makers (Split reps between arms) •12 Burpees •500-meter Run •36 Air Squats •12 Hand-release push-ups					
3	10 Rounds for Time of: •250 meter Run •15 Deadlift Burpee Dumbbells					
4	3 Rounds for Time of: •1,000-meter Run •30 Dumbbell Squat Cleans					
5	10 Rounds for Time of: •10 Dumbbell man-makers (Split reps between arms) •20 Dumbbell Deadlifts					

		Day 1	Day 2	Day 3	Day 4	Day 5
WORKOUTS		Reps / Time / Weight	Reps / Time / Weight	Reps / Time / Weight	Reps / Time / Weight	Reps / Time / Weight
6	•30 Burpees •30 Dumbbell Deadlifts •30 Burpees •30 Dumbbell Cleans •30 Burpees •30 Single-Arm Dumbbell Strict Presses (Split reps between arms) •30 Burpees •30 Dumbbell Push Presses •30 Burpees •30 Dumbbell Thrusters •30 Burpees •30 Dumbbell Swings •30 Burpees •30 Dumbbell Sumo Deadlift High-Pulls •30 Burpees •30 Dumbbell Snatches (Left Hand) •30 Burpees •30 Dumbbell Snatches (Right Hand) •30 Burpees •30 Dumbbell Man Makers (Split reps between arms)					
7	1-3-5-7-9-11-13-15 Reps for Time of: •Dumbbell Clusters (Dumbbell Clean + Dumbbell Thrusters) •100-meter run					
8	•100 Dumbbell Hang Clean Thrusters					
9	21-12-9 Reps for Time of: •Dumbbell Thrusters •Air Squats •Burpees					

	WORKOUTS	Day 6 Reps / Time / Weight	Day 7 Reps / Time / Weight	Day 8 Reps / Time / Weight	Day 9 Reps / Time / Weight	Day 10 Reps / Time / Weight
6	•30 Burpees •30 Dumbbell Deadlifts •30 Burpees •30 Dumbbell Cleans •30 Burpees •30 Single-Arm Dumbbell Strict Presses (Split reps between arms) •30 Burpees •30 Dumbbell Push Presses •30 Burpees •30 Dumbbell Thrusters •30 Burpees •30 Dumbbell Swings •30 Burpees •30 Dumbbell Sumo Deadlift High-Pulls •30 Burpees •30 Dumbbell Snatches (Left Hand) •30 Burpees •30 Dumbbell Snatches (Right Hand) •30 Burpees •30 Dumbbell Man Makers (Split reps between arms)					
7	1-3-5-7-9-11-13-15 Reps for Time of: •Dumbbell Clusters (Dumbbell Clean + Dumbbell Thrusters) •100-meter run					
8	•100 Dumbbell Hang Clean Thrusters					
9	21-12-9 Reps for Time of: •Dumbbell Thrusters •Air Squats •Burpees					

	WORKOUTS	Day 1	Day 2	Day 3	Day 4	Day 5
		Reps / Time / Weight	Reps / Time / Weight	Reps / Time / Weight	Reps / Time / Weight	Reps / Time / Weight
10	5 Rounds for Time of: •10 Dumbbell Power Snatches (Per arm) •20 Dumbbell Thrusters •20 Push-ups					
11	11-10-9-8-7-6-5-4-3-2-1 Reps of: •Dumbbell Snatches (Per arm) •Hand-release push-ups					
12	•Every minute on the minute for 3 minutes: •16 Dumbbell Rows (Split reps between arms) •10 Push-Ups •Every minute on the minute for 3 minutes: •14 Dumbbell Rows (Split reps between arms) •10 Push-Ups •Every minute on the minute for 3 minutes: •12 Dumbbell Rows •10 Push-Ups Then, As many rounds as possible in 3 minutes of: •Dumbbell Rows					
13	4 Rounds for Time of: •400 meter Run •40 Dumbbell Deadlifts •40 Sit-Ups					

WORKOUTS		Day 6 Reps / Time / Weight	Day 7 Reps / Time / Weight	Day 8 Reps / Time / Weight	Day 9 Reps / Time / Weight	Day 10 Reps / Time / Weight
10	5 Rounds for Time of: • 10 Dumbbell Power Snatches (Per arm) • 20 Dumbbell Thrusters • 20 Push-ups					
11	11-10-9-8-7-6-5-4-3-2-1 Reps of: • Dumbbell Snatches (Per arm) • Hand-release push-ups					
12	• Every minute on the minute for 3 minutes: • 16 Dumbbell Rows (Split reps between arms) • 10 Push-Ups • Every minute on the minute for 3 minutes: • 14 Dumbbell Rows (Split reps between arms) • 10 Push-Ups • Every minute on the minute for 3 minutes: • 12 Dumbbell Rows • 10 Push-Ups Then, As many rounds as possible in 3 minutes of: • Dumbbell Rows					
13	4 Rounds for Time of: • 400 meter Run • 40 Dumbbell Deadlifts • 40 Sit-Ups					

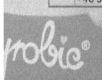

	WORKOUTS	Day 1 Reps / Time / Weight	Day 2 Reps / Time / Weight	Day 3 Reps / Time / Weight	Day 4 Reps / Time / Weight	Day 5 Reps / Time / Weight
14	•50 Dumbbell Power Snatches (Split reps between arms) •25-meter Dumbbell Overhead Walking Lunges (Per arm) •40 Dumbbell Overhead Squats (Alternate arms every 10 reps) •25-meter Dumbbell Overhead Walking Lunges (Per arm) •30 Dumbbell Hang Clean-and-Jerks (Alternate arms every 5 reps) •25-meter Dumbbell Overhead Walking Lunges (Per arm) •20 Dumbbell Squat Cleans •25-meter Dumbbell Overhead Walking Lunges (Per arm)					
15	•100 Double Dumbbell Ground-to-Overhead					
16	•40 Dumbbell Thrusters •1000-meter Run •40 Burpees					
17	3 Rounds for Time of: •30 Dumbbell Bicep Curls (Split reps between arms) •30 Dumbbell Strict Presses (Split reps between arms) •30 Dumbbell Lateral Raises (Split reps between arms) •30 Dumbbell Hammer Curls •30 Dumbbell Upright Rows •30 Dumbbell Push Presses •30 Dumbbell Bicep Curls					

	WORKOUTS	Day 6 Reps / Time / Weight	Day 7 Reps / Time / Weight	Day 8 Reps / Time / Weight	Day 9 Reps / Time / Weight	Day 10 Reps / Time / Weight
14	•50 Dumbbell Power Snatches (Split reps between arms) •25-meter Dumbbell Overhead Walking Lunges (Per arm) •40 Dumbbell Overhead Squats (Alternate arms every 10 reps) •25-meter Dumbbell Overhead Walking Lunges (Per arm) •30 Dumbbell Hang Clean-and-Jerks (Alternate arms every 5 reps) •25-meter Dumbbell Overhead Walking Lunges (Per arm) •20 Dumbbell Squat Cleans •25-meter Dumbbell Overhead Walking Lunges (Per arm)					
15	•100 Double Dumbbell Ground-to-Overhead					
16	•40 Dumbbell Thrusters •1000-meter Run •40 Burpees					
17	3 Rounds for Time of: •30 Dumbbell Bicep Curls (Split reps between arms) •30 Dumbbell Strict Presses (Split reps between arms) •30 Dumbbell Lateral Raises (Split reps between arms) •30 Dumbbell Hammer Curls •30 Dumbbell Upright Rows •30 Dumbbell Push Presses •30 Dumbbell Bicep Curls					

	WORKOUTS	Day 1 Reps / Time / Weight	Day 2 Reps / Time / Weight	Day 3 Reps / Time / Weight	Day 4 Reps / Time / Weight	Day 5 Reps / Time / Weight
18	2 Rounds for Time of: •30 Dumbbell Squats •30 Burpees •300-meter Run •30 Dumbbell Push Presses •30 Lateral Jumps Over Dumbbells •30 Dumbbell Power Cleans •30 Dumbbell Lunges					
19	•30 Dumbbell Devil Presses •60 Dumbbell Thrusters •90 Burpees					
20	•11 Dumbbell Snatches (Left arm) •11 Dumbbell Overhead Lunges (Left arm) •11 Dumbbell Snatches (Right arm) •11 Dumbbell Overhead Lunges (Right arm) •11 Dumbbell Power Cleans (Left arm) •11 Dumbbell Squats (Left arm) •11 Dumbbell Power Cleans (Right arm) •11 Dumbbell Squats (Right arm)					
21	10 Rounds for Time of: •1 Dumbbell Push-Up •1 Dumbbell Plank Row (Right-Arm) •1 Dumbbell Plank Row (Left-Arm) •1 Dumbbell Clean •1 Dumbbell Front Squat •1 Dumbbell Push Press •1 Dumbbell Overhead Reverse Lunge (Each leg) •200-meter Run					

	Day 6	Day 7	Day 8	Day 9	Day 10
WORKOUTS	Reps / Time / Weight	Reps / Time / Weight	Reps / Time / Weight	Reps / Time / Weight	Reps / Time / Weight
18 2 Rounds for Time of: •30 Dumbbell Squats •30 Burpees •300-meter Run •30 Dumbbell Push Presses •30 Lateral Jumps Over Dumbbells •30 Dumbbell Power Cleans •30 Dumbbell Lunges					
19 •30 Dumbbell Devil Presses •60 Dumbbell Thrusters •90 Burpees					
20 •11 Dumbbell Snatches (Left arm) •11 Dumbbell Overhead Lunges (Left arm) •11 Dumbbell Snatches (Right arm) •11 Dumbbell Overhead Lunges (Right arm) •11 Dumbbell Power Cleans (Left arm) •11 Dumbbell Squats (Left arm) •11 Dumbbell Power Cleans (Right arm) •11 Dumbbell Squats (Right arm)					
21 10 Rounds for Time of: •1 Dumbbell Push-Up •1 Dumbbell Plank Row (Right-Arm) •1 Dumbbell Plank Row (Left-Arm) •1 Dumbbell Clean •1 Dumbbell Front Squat •1 Dumbbell Push Press •1 Dumbbell Overhead Reverse Lunge (Each leg) •200-meter Run					

	WORKOUTS	Day 1 Reps / Time / Weight	Day 2 Reps / Time / Weight	Day 3 Reps / Time / Weight	Day 4 Reps / Time / Weight	Day 5 Reps / Time / Weight
22	•500-meter Run •25 Dumbbell Clean and Presses •500-meter Run •25 Dumbbell Thrusters •500-meter Run •25 Dumbbell Burpees and Presses •500-meter Run					
23	•1,000-meter run •Max Dumbbell Thrusters •1,000-meter run					
24	•1,500-meter Run Then, 5 Rounds for Time of: •20 Burpees •10 Dumbbell Snatches (Per arm) •20 Dumbbell Thrusters •20 Dumbbell Devil Presses Finally, perform: •500-meter Run					
25	10 Rounds for Time of: •30 Dumbbell Lunges •5 Dumbbell Devil Presses •20 Air Squats •20 Push-ups •100 Burpees					

	WORKOUTS	Day 6 Reps / Time / Weight	Day 7 Reps / Time / Weight	Day 8 Reps / Time / Weight	Day 9 Reps / Time / Weight	Day 10 Reps / Time / Weight
22	•500-meter Run •25 Dumbbell Clean and Presses •500-meter Run •25 Dumbbell Thrusters •500-meter Run •25 Dumbbell Burpees and Presses •500-meter Run					
23	•1,000-meter run •Max Dumbbell Thrusters •1,000-meter run					
24	•1,500-meter Run Then, 5 Rounds for Time of: •20 Burpees •10 Dumbbell Snatches (Per arm) •20 Dumbbell Thrusters •20 Dumbbell Devil Presses Finally, perform: •500-meter Run					
25	10 Rounds for Time of: •30 Dumbbell Lunges •5 Dumbbell Devil Presses •20 Air Squats •20 Push-ups •100 Burpees					

	Day 1 Reps / Time / Weight	Day 2 Reps / Time / Weight	Day 3 Reps / Time / Weight	Day 4 Reps / Time / Weight	Day 5 Reps / Time / Weight
WORKOUTS					
26	•21 Burpees •1 Round of "Dumbbell DT" •18 Burpees •1 Round of "Dumbbell DT" •15 Burpees •1 Round of "Dumbbell DT" •12 Burpees •1 Round of "Dumbbell DT" •21 Air Squats Hops Over Dumbbell •1 Round of "Dumbbell DT" •18 Air Squats Hops Over Dumbbell •1 Round of "Dumbbell DT" •15 Air Squats Hops Over Dumbbell •1 Round of "Dumbbell DT" •12 Air Squat Hops Over Dumbbell •1 Round of "Dumbbell DT" 1 Round of "Dumbbell DT"				
27	•15 Dumbbell Sit-Ups •20 Russian Twists with Dumbbell •10 Dumbbell Push Presses •10 Dumbbell Squats •10 V-Ups				
28	•3 Rounds for Time of: •10 Push-ups •12 Dumbbell Hang Snatches (Split reps between arms) •14 Cossack Squats •3 Rounds for Time of: •10 Burpees •12 Dumbbell Hang Snatches (Split reps between arms) •14 Mantis Get-ups				

	WORKOUTS	Day 6 Reps / Time / Weight	Day 7 Reps / Time / Weight	Day 8 Reps / Time / Weight	Day 9 Reps / Time / Weight	Day 10 Reps / Time / Weight
26	•21 Burpees •1 Round of "Dumbbell DT" •18 Burpees •1 Round of "Dumbbell DT" •15 Burpees •1 Round of "Dumbbell DT" •12 Burpees •1 Round of "Dumbbell DT" •21 Air Squats Hops Over Dumbbell •1 Round of "Dumbbell DT" •18 Air Squats Hops Over Dumbbell •1 Round of "Dumbbell DT" •15 Air Squats Hops Over Dumbbell •1 Round of "Dumbbell DT" •12 Air Squat Hops Over Dumbbell •1 Round of "Dumbbell DT" 1 Round of "Dumbbell DT"					
27	•15 Dumbbell Sit-Ups •20 Russian Twists with Dumbbell •10 Dumbbell Push Presses •10 Dumbbell Squats •10 V-Ups					
28	•3 Rounds for Time of: •10 Push-ups •12 Dumbbell Hang Snatches (Split reps between arms) •14 Cossack Squats •3 Rounds for Time of: •10 Burpees •12 Dumbbell Hang Snatches (Split reps between arms) •14 Mantis Get-ups					

	WORKOUTS	Day 1 Reps / Time / Weight	Day 2 Reps / Time / Weight	Day 3 Reps / Time / Weight	Day 4 Reps / Time / Weight	Day 5 Reps / Time / Weight
29	•1,000-meter Run •50 Dumbbell Devil Presses •1,000-meter Run					
30	•12 Dumbbell Power Snatches (Split reps between arms) •12 Dumbbell Renegade Rows (Split reps between arms) •12 Dumbbell Power Cleans					
31	•3 Rounds for Time of: •20 Dumbbell Lunges (Alternate legs) •20 Dumbbell Snatches (Alternate arms)					
32	•30 Burpees Over a Dumbbell •3 Rounds for Time of: •30 Dumbbell Hang Clean-and-Jerks (Alternate arms) •30 Dumbbell Squats					
33	3 Rounds for Time of: •12 Dumbbell Sumo Squats •10 Arnold Press (Both arms) •10 Dumbbell Suitcase Lunges (Split reps between legs) •10 Dumbbell Sit Up with Press •12 Half-Burpees Over Dumbbell					

	WORKOUTS	Day 6	Day 7	Day 8	Day 9	Day 10
		Reps / Time / Weight	Reps / Time / Weight	Reps / Time / Weight	Reps / Time / Weight	Reps / Time / Weight
29	•1,000-meter Run •50 Dumbbell Devil Presses •1,000-meter Run					
30	•12 Dumbbell Power Snatches (Split reps between arms) •12 Dumbbell Renegade Rows (Split reps between arms) •12 Dumbbell Power Cleans					
31	•3 Rounds for Time of: •20 Dumbbell Lunges (Alternate legs) •20 Dumbbell Snatches (Alternate arms)					
32	•30 Burpees Over a Dumbbell •3 Rounds for Time of: •30 Dumbbell Hang Clean-and-Jerks (Alternate arms) •30 Dumbbell Squats					
33	3 Rounds for Time of: •12 Dumbbell Sumo Squats •10 Arnold Press (Both arms) •10 Dumbbell Suitcase Lunges (Split reps between legs) •10 Dumbbell Sit Up with Press •12 Half-Burpees Over Dumbbell					

	WORKOUTS	Day 1 Reps / Time / Weight	Day 2 Reps / Time / Weight	Day 3 Reps / Time / Weight	Day 4 Reps / Time / Weight	Day 5 Reps / Time / Weight
34	•500-meter Run •30 Dumbbell Squats •40 Burpees •50 Dumbbell Push Jerks •15 Dumbbell Squats •20 Burpees •25 Dumbbell Push Jerks					
35	For Time of: •100 Dumbbell Hang Clean Thrusters •5 Push-ups to start, and at the end of each minute					
36	As many rounds as possible in 17 minutes of: •7 Dumbbell Goblet Thrusters •7 Dumbbell Power Snatches (Each arm) •7 Burpees					
37	As many rounds as possible in 16 minutes of: •6 Burpees •10 Hand-Release Push-Up •14 Dumbbell Goblet Squat					
38	•20 Air Squat Hops Over Dumbbell •40 Dumbbell Shoulder to Overhead (Split reps between arms) •20 Air Squat Hops Over Dumbbell •30 Dumbbell Squat Cleans (Split reps between arms) •20 Air Squat Hops Over Dumbbell •20 Dumbbell Thrusters •20 Air Squat Hops Over Dumbbell •10 Dumbbell Clusters •20 Air Squat Hops Over Dumbbell					

	WORKOUTS	Day 6 Reps / Time / Weight	Day 7 Reps / Time / Weight	Day 8 Reps / Time / Weight	Day 9 Reps / Time / Weight	Day 10 Reps / Time / Weight
34	•500-meter Run •30 Dumbbell Squats •40 Burpees •50 Dumbbell Push Jerks •15 Dumbbell Squats •20 Burpees •25 Dumbbell Push Jerks					
35	For Time of: •100 Dumbbell Hang Clean Thrusters •5 Push-ups to start, and at the end of each minute					
36	As many rounds as possible in 17 minutes of: •7 Dumbbell Goblet Thrusters •7 Dumbbell Power Snatches (Each arm) •7 Burpees					
37	As many rounds as possible in 16 minutes of: •6 Burpees •10 Hand-Release Push-Up •14 Dumbbell Goblet Squat					
38	•20 Air Squat Hops Over Dumbbell •40 Dumbbell Shoulder to Overhead (Split reps between arms) •20 Air Squat Hops Over Dumbbell •30 Dumbbell Squat Cleans (Split reps between arms) •20 Air Squat Hops Over Dumbbell •20 Dumbbell Thrusters •20 Air Squat Hops Over Dumbbell •10 Dumbbell Clusters •20 Air Squat Hops Over Dumbbell					

	WORKOUTS	Day 1	Day 2	Day 3	Day 4	Day 5
		Reps / Time / Weight	Reps / Time / Weight	Reps / Time / Weight	Reps / Time / Weight	Reps / Time / Weight
39	•30 Burpees •30 Dumbbell Clean and Jerks •30 Dumbbell Snatches (Split reps between arms) •30 Burpees					
40	•30 Air Squat Hops Over Dumbbell •40 Dumbbell Shoulder to Overhead •30 Air Squat Hops Over Dumbbell •30 Dumbbell Squat Cleans •30 Air Squat Hops Over Dumbbell •20 Dumbbell Thrusters •30 Air Squat Hops Over Dumbbell •10 Dumbbell Clusters (Dumbbell Clean + Dumbbell Thrusters) •30 Air Squat Hops Over Dumbbell					
41	•10 Devil Presses •20 Dumbbell Lunges (Alternate legs) •30 Dumbbell Push Presses •40 Sit-Ups					
42	•5 Rounds for Time of: •9 Devil Presses •20 Dumbbell Lunges (Alternate legs) •9 Dumbbell Push Presses •20 Sit-Ups					

	WORKOUTS	Day 6 Reps / Time / Weight	Day 7 Reps / Time / Weight	Day 8 Reps / Time / Weight	Day 9 Reps / Time / Weight	Day 10 Reps / Time / Weight
39	•30 Burpees •30 Dumbbell Clean and Jerks •30 Dumbbell Snatches (Split reps between arms) •30 Burpees					
40	•30 Air Squat Hops Over Dumbbell •40 Dumbbell Shoulder to Overhead •30 Air Squat Hops Over Dumbbell •30 Dumbbell Squat Cleans •30 Air Squat Hops Over Dumbbell •20 Dumbbell Thrusters •30 Air Squat Hops Over Dumbbell •10 Dumbbell Clusters (Dumbbell Clean + Dumbbell Thrusters) •30 Air Squat Hops Over Dumbbell					
41	•10 Devil Presses •20 Dumbbell Lunges (Alternate legs) •30 Dumbbell Push Presses •40 Sit-Ups					
42	•5 Rounds for Time of: •9 Devil Presses •20 Dumbbell Lunges (Alternate legs) •9 Dumbbell Push Presses •20 Sit-Ups					

	WORKOUTS	Day 1 Reps / Time / Weight	Day 2 Reps / Time / Weight	Day 3 Reps / Time / Weight	Day 4 Reps / Time / Weight	Day 5 Reps / Time / Weight
43	•1000-meter Run •2 Rounds for Time of: •12 Dumbbell Deadlifts •12 Dumbbell Swings •12 Dumbbell Thrusters					
44	•12 Rounds for Time of: •10 Dumbbell Hang Squat Cleans •10 Dumbbell Power Snatches (Split reps between arms)					
45	•20 Burpees •21 Dumbbell Snatches (Each arm) •12 Dumbbell Thrusters •20 Burpees •21 Dumbbell Snatches (Each arm) •12 Dumbbell Thrusters					
46	•3 Dumbbell Hang Clean •4 Dumbbell Squats •5 Dumbbell Push Jerk •6 Bent Over Rows •7 Burpees •8 Dumbbell Thrusters •9 Dumbbell Deadlifts •10 Dumbbell Snatches (Split reps between arms) •11 Dumbbell Swings •12 Dumbbell Snatch To Reverse Lunge (Split reps between arms) •13 Dumbbell Devils Press •1000-meter Run					

		Day 6	Day 7	Day 8	Day 9	Day 10
	WORKOUTS	Reps / Time / Weight	Reps / Time / Weight	Reps / Time / Weight	Reps / Time / Weight	Reps / Time / Weight
43	•1000-meter Run •2 Rounds for Time of: •12 Dumbbell Deadlifts •12 Dumbbell Swings •12 Dumbbell Thrusters					
44	•12 Rounds for Time of: •10 Dumbbell Hang Squat Cleans •10 Dumbbell Power Snatches (Split reps between arms)					
45	•20 Burpees •21 Dumbbell Snatches (Each arm) •12 Dumbbell Thrusters •20 Burpees •21 Dumbbell Snatches (Each arm) •12 Dumbbell Thrusters					
46	•3 Dumbbell Hang Clean •4 Dumbbell Squats •5 Dumbbell Push Jerk •6 Bent Over Rows •7 Burpees •8 Dumbbell Thrusters •9 Dumbbell Deadlifts •10 Dumbbell Snatches (Split reps between arms) •11 Dumbbell Swings •12 Dumbbell Snatch To Reverse Lunge (Split reps between arms) •13 Dumbbell Devils Press •1000-meter Run					

	WORKOUTS	Day 1	Day 2	Day 3	Day 4	Day 5
		Reps / Time / Weight	Reps / Time / Weight	Reps / Time / Weight	Reps / Time / Weight	Reps / Time / Weight
47	•15 Dumbbell Devil Presses •30 Air Squats •12 Dumbbell Devil Presses •30 Air Squats •9 Dumbbell Devil Presses •30 Air Squats •6 Dumbbell Devil Presses •30 Air Squats •3 Dumbbell Devil Presses •30 Air Squats					
48	•50 Air Squats •50 Dumbbell Snatches (Alternate arms) •40 Air Squats •40 Dumbbell Snatches (Alternate arms) •30 Air Squats •30 Dumbbell Snatches (Alternate arms) •20 Air Squats •20 Dumbbell Snatches (Alternate arms) •10 Air Squats •10 Dumbbell Snatches (Alternate arms)					
49	•2-minute Max Dumbbell Renegade Rows •2-minute Max Push-Ups •2-minute Max Mountain Climbers •2-minute Max Air Squats •2-minute Max Dumbbell Power Snatches (Alternate arms)					
50	•5 Rounds for Time of: •10 Single-Arm Dumbbell Floor Press (Split reps between arms) •14 Russian Twists with Dumbbell •18 Dumbbell Windmill (Split reps between arms) •22 Dumbbell Sit-Up					

	WORKOUTS	Day 6 Reps / Time / Weight	Day 7 Reps / Time / Weight	Day 8 Reps / Time / Weight	Day 9 Reps / Time / Weight	Day 10 Reps / Time / Weight
47	•15 Dumbbell Devil Presses •30 Air Squats •12 Dumbbell Devil Presses •30 Air Squats •9 Dumbbell Devil Presses •30 Air Squats •6 Dumbbell Devil Presses •30 Air Squats •3 Dumbbell Devil Presses •30 Air Squats					
48	•50 Air Squats •50 Dumbbell Snatches (Alternate arms) •40 Air Squats •40 Dumbbell Snatches (Alternate arms) •30 Air Squats •30 Dumbbell Snatches (Alternate arms) •20 Air Squats •20 Dumbbell Snatches (Alternate arms) •10 Air Squats •10 Dumbbell Snatches (Alternate arms)					
49	•2-minute Max Dumbbell Renegade Rows •2-minute Max Push-Ups •2-minute Max Mountain Climbers •2-minute Max Air Squats •2-minute Max Dumbbell Power Snatches (Alternate arms)					
50	•5 Rounds for Time of: •10 Single-Arm Dumbbell Floor Press (Split reps between arms) •14 Russian Twists with Dumbbell •18 Dumbbell Windmill (Split reps between arms) •22 Dumbbell Sit-Up					

		Day 1	Day 2	Day 3	Day 4	Day 5
WORKOUTS		Reps / Time / Weight	Reps / Time / Weight	Reps / Time / Weight	Reps / Time / Weight	Reps / Time / Weight
51	•4 Dumbbell Renegade Rows •16 Dumbbell Snatches (Alternate arms) •24 Lateral Hops Over Dumbbell •4 Dumbbell Renegade Rows •16 Dumbbell Snatches (Alternate arms) •24 Lateral Hops Over Dumbbell					
52	As many rounds as possible in 26 minutes of: •6 Dumbbell Devil Presses •6 Burpees Over Dumbbells •6 Dumbbell Thrusters					
53	As many reps as possible in 10 minutes of: •10 Dumbbell Thrusters •10 Burpee					
54	•100 Dumbbell Thrusters •1 Burpee Keep adding 1 Burpee after every minute					
55	•30 Dumbbell Farmer's Carry (Alternate Lunges) •30 Push-Ups •30 Dumbbell Bent Over Rows •20 Dumbbell Farmer's Carry (Alternate Lunges) •20 Push-Ups •20 Dumbbell Bent Over Rows •10 Dumbbell Farmer's Carry (Alternate Lunges) •10 Push-Ups •10 Dumbbell Bent Over Rows					

	WORKOUTS	Day 6 Reps / Time / Weight	Day 7 Reps / Time / Weight	Day 8 Reps / Time / Weight	Day 9 Reps / Time / Weight	Day 10 Reps / Time / Weight
51	•4 Dumbbell Renegade Rows •16 Dumbbell Snatches (Alternate arms) •24 Lateral Hops Over Dumbbell •4 Dumbbell Renegade Rows •16 Dumbbell Snatches (Alternate arms) •24 Lateral Hops Over Dumbbell					
52	As many rounds as possible in 26 minutes of: •6 Dumbbell Devil Presses •6 Burpees Over Dumbbells •6 Dumbbell Thrusters					
53	As many reps as possible in 10 minutes of: •10 Dumbbell Thrusters •10 Burpee					
54	•100 Dumbbell Thrusters •1 Burpee Keep adding 1 Burpee after every minute					
55	•30 Dumbbell Farmer's Carry (Alternate Lunges) •30 Push-Ups •30 Dumbbell Bent Over Rows •20 Dumbbell Farmer's Carry (Alternate Lunges) •20 Push-Ups •20 Dumbbell Bent Over Rows •10 Dumbbell Farmer's Carry (Alternate Lunges) •10 Push-Ups •10 Dumbbell Bent Over Rows					

	WORKOUTS	Day 1 Reps / Time / Weight	Day 2 Reps / Time / Weight	Day 3 Reps / Time / Weight	Day 4 Reps / Time / Weight	Day 5 Reps / Time / Weight
56	As many reps as possible in 10 minutes of: •10 Dumbbell Deadlifts •10 Renegade Row (Alternate arms) with Pushup					
57	5 Rounds for Time of: •30 Dumbbell Hang Squat Cleans •20 Burpees over Dumbbell •10 Push-ups					
58	•20 Alternate Jumping Lunges •20 Dumbbell Sumo Deadlifts •20 Dumbbell Push Presses •15 Alternate Jumping Lunges •15 Dumbbell Sumo Deadlifts •15 Dumbbell Push Presses •10 Alternate Jumping Lunges •10 Dumbbell Sumo Deadlifts •10 Dumbbell Push Presses					
59	For Time of: •40 Dumbbell Goblet Squats •50 Push-Ups •60 Air Squats •50 Push-Ups •40 Dumbbell Goblet Squats					
60	•60-second Max Up-Downs •60-second Max Dumbbell Hang Power Cleans •60-second max Renegade Rows					

	WORKOUTS	Day 6 Reps / Time / Weight	Day 7 Reps / Time / Weight	Day 8 Reps / Time / Weight	Day 9 Reps / Time / Weight	Day 10 Reps / Time / Weight
56	As many reps as possible in 10 minutes of: •10 Dumbbell Deadlifts •10 Renegade Row (Alternate arms) with Pushup					
57	5 Rounds for Time of: •30 Dumbbell Hang Squat Cleans •20 Burpees over Dumbbell •10 Push-ups					
58	•20 Alternate Jumping Lunges •20 Dumbbell Sumo Deadlifts •20 Dumbbell Push Presses •15 Alternate Jumping Lunges •15 Dumbbell Sumo Deadlifts •15 Dumbbell Push Presses •10 Alternate Jumping Lunges •10 Dumbbell Sumo Deadlifts •10 Dumbbell Push Presses					
59	For Time of: •40 Dumbbell Goblet Squats •50 Push-Ups •60 Air Squats •50 Push-Ups •40 Dumbbell Goblet Squats					
60	•60-second Max Up-Downs •60-second Max Dumbbell Hang Power Cleans •60-second max Renegade Rows					

	WORKOUTS	Day 1 Reps / Time / Weight	Day 2 Reps / Time / Weight	Day 3 Reps / Time / Weight	Day 4 Reps / Time / Weight	Day 5 Reps / Time / Weight
61	•11-10-9-8-7-6-5-4-3-2-1 Dumbbell Squat Cleans •11 Burpees					
62	•5 Rounds for Time of: •20 Dumbbell Hang Power Cleans •20 Renegade Row (Alternate arms) with Pushup					
63	As many rounds as possible in 20 minutes of: •10 Dumbbell Hang Snatches (Alternate arms) •20 Burpees •30 Push-ups					
64	21-15-9 Reps for Time of: •Dumbbell Ground-to-Overheads •Push-Ups 9-15-21 Reps for Time of: •Dumbbell Swings •Push-Ups					
65	•For Time of 30-20-10 Reps for: •Dumbbell Hang Squat Thrusters •Burpees over Dumbbell •V-ups					
66	As many rounds as possible in 25 minutes of: •500-meter Run •25 Dumbbell Power Cleans					

	WORKOUTS	Day 6 Reps / Time / Weight	Day 7 Reps / Time / Weight	Day 8 Reps / Time / Weight	Day 9 Reps / Time / Weight	Day 10 Reps / Time / Weight
61	•11-10-9-8-7-6-5-4-3-2-1 Dumbbell Squat Cleans •11 Burpees					
62	•5 Rounds for Time of: •20 Dumbbell Hang Power Cleans •20 Renegade Row (Alternate arms) with Pushup					
63	As many rounds as possible in 20 minutes of: •10 Dumbbell Hang Snatches (Alternate arms) •20 Burpees •30 Push-ups					
64	21-15-9 Reps for Time of: •Dumbbell Ground-to-Overheads •Push-Ups 9-15-21 Reps for Time of: •Dumbbell Swings •Push-Ups					
65	•For Time of 30-20-10 Reps for: •Dumbbell Hang Squat Thrusters •Burpees over Dumbbell •V-ups					
66	As many rounds as possible in 25 minutes of: •500-meter Run •25 Dumbbell Power Cleans					

	WORKOUTS	Day 1 Reps / Time / Weight	Day 2 Reps / Time / Weight	Day 3 Reps / Time / Weight	Day 4 Reps / Time / Weight	Day 5 Reps / Time / Weight
67	•2,000-meter Run •21 Air Squats •5 Burpees •21 Dumbbell Shoulder Presses •5 Burpees •21 Dumbbell Lunges •5 Burpees •21 Bicep Curls •5 Burpees •2,000-meter Run •9 Push-Ups					
68	For Time for 45-30-15 Reps of: •Dumbbell Thrusters •Push-ups					
69	•50 Dumbbell Lunges (Alternate legs) •40 Sit-Ups •30 Burpees •20 Hand Release Push-Ups •10 Dumbbell Deadlifts •20 Hand Release Push-Ups •30 Burpees •40 Sit-Ups •50 Dumbbell Lunges (Alternate legs)					
70	10 Rounds for Time of: •10 Dumbbell Goblet Squats •10 Dumbbell Power Snatches (Alternate arms) •10 Dumbbell Overhead Squats (Alternate arms)					
71	5 Rounds for Time of: •5 Dumbbell Thrusters •5 Dumbbell Sumo Deadlift High Pulls •5 Dumbbell Hang Cleans •5 Burpees					

	WORKOUTS	Day 6 Reps / Time / Weight	Day 7 Reps / Time / Weight	Day 8 Reps / Time / Weight	Day 9 Reps / Time / Weight	Day 10 Reps / Time / Weight
67	•2,000-meter Run •21 Air Squats •5 Burpees •21 Dumbbell Shoulder Presses •5 Burpees •21 Dumbbell Lunges •5 Burpees •21 Bicep Curls •5 Burpees •2,000-meter Run •9 Push-Ups					
68	For Time for 45-30-15 Reps of: •Dumbbell Thrusters •Push-ups					
69	•50 Dumbbell Lunges (Alternate legs) •40 Sit-Ups •30 Burpees •20 Hand Release Push-Ups •10 Dumbbell Deadlifts •20 Hand Release Push-Ups •30 Burpees •40 Sit-Ups •50 Dumbbell Lunges (Alternate legs)					
70	10 Rounds for Time of: •10 Dumbbell Goblet Squats •10 Dumbbell Power Snatches (Alternate arms) •10 Dumbbell Overhead Squats (Alternate arms)					
71	5 Rounds for Time of: •5 Dumbbell Thrusters •5 Dumbbell Sumo Deadlift High Pulls •5 Dumbbell Hang Cleans •5 Burpees					

	WORKOUTS	Day 1 Reps / Time / Weight	Day 2 Reps / Time / Weight	Day 3 Reps / Time / Weight	Day 4 Reps / Time / Weight	Day 5 Reps / Time / Weight
72	•10 Dumbbell Power Snatches (Left-Arm) •50 Jumping Jacks •10 Dumbbell Power Snatches (Right-Arm) •50 Jumping Jacks •10 Dumbbell Renegade Rows (Left-Arm) •50 Jumping Jacks •10 Dumbbell Renegade Rows (Right-Arm)					
73	•As many rounds as possible in 24 minutes of: •24 Overhead Dumbbell Lunges •12 Burpees •6 Push-ups					
74	•3 Rounds for Time of: •60 Lunges (Alternate legs) •50 Air squats •40 Sit-ups •30 Push-ups •20 Burpees •10 Dumbbell Thrusters					
75	•11 Dumbbell Deadlifts •11 Spider-Man Push-Ups •10 Dumbbell Deadlifts •10 Spider-Man Push-Ups •9 Dumbbell Deadlifts •9 Diamond Push-Ups •8 Dumbbell Deadlifts •8 Spider-Man Push-Ups •7 Dumbbell Deadlifts •7 Diamond Push-Ups •6 Dumbbell Deadlifts •6 Spider-Man Push-Ups •5 Dumbbell Deadlifts •5 Diamond Push-Ups •4 Dumbbell Deadlifts •4 Spider-Man Push-Ups •3 Dumbbell Deadlifts •3 Diamond Push-Ups •2 Dumbbell Deadlifts •2 Spider-Man Push-Ups •1 Dumbbell Deadlift •1 Diamond Push-Up					

	WORKOUTS	Day 6 Reps / Time / Weight	Day 7 Reps / Time / Weight	Day 8 Reps / Time / Weight	Day 9 Reps / Time / Weight	Day 10 Reps / Time / Weight
72	•10 Dumbbell Power Snatches (Left-Arm) •50 Jumping Jacks •10 Dumbbell Power Snatches (Right-Arm) •50 Jumping Jacks •10 Dumbbell Renegade Rows (Left-Arm) •50 Jumping Jacks •10 Dumbbell Renegade Rows (Right-Arm)					
73	•As many rounds as possible in 24 minutes of: •24 Overhead Dumbbell Lunges •12 Burpees •6 Push-ups					
74	•3 Rounds for Time of: •60 Lunges (Alternate legs) •50 Air squats •40 Sit-ups •30 Push-ups •20 Burpees •10 Dumbbell Thrusters					
75	•11 Dumbbell Deadlifts •11 Spider-Man Push-Ups •10 Dumbbell Deadlifts •10 Spider-Man Push-Ups •9 Dumbbell Deadlifts •9 Diamond Push-Ups •8 Dumbbell Deadlifts •8 Spider-Man Push-Ups •7 Dumbbell Deadlifts •7 Diamond Push-Ups •6 Dumbbell Deadlifts •6 Spider-Man Push-Ups •5 Dumbbell Deadlifts •5 Diamond Push-Ups •4 Dumbbell Deadlifts •4 Spider-Man Push-Ups •3 Dumbbell Deadlifts •3 Diamond Push-Ups •2 Dumbbell Deadlifts •2 Spider-Man Push-Ups •1 Dumbbell Deadlift •1 Diamond Push-Up					

	Day 1	Day 2	Day 3	Day 4	Day 5
WORKOUTS	Reps / Time / Weight	Reps / Time / Weight	Reps / Time / Weight	Reps / Time / Weight	Reps / Time / Weight
76 •5 Rounds for Time of: •20 Dumbbell Floor Press •20 Dumbbell Sumo Squats •20 Dumbbell Thrusters •20 Push-ups					
77 As many reps as possible in 15 minutes of: •10 Dumbbell Push-up with Row (Alternate arms) •10 Dumbbell Snatches •10 Dumbbell Squats					
78 •50 Dumbbell Strict Presses •50 Dumbbell Pull-Overs •50 Dumbbell Bent Over Rows					
79 •50 Dumbbell Man-Makers •1,000-meter Run •25 Dumbbell Devil Presses					
80 For Time of: •1,000-meter Run Then, 3 Rounds for Time of: •8 Dumbbell Burpees to Presses •100-meter Farmer's Carry •8 Dual Dumbbell Overhead Reverse Lunge (Alternate legs) •100 Air Squats Finally, perform: •1,000-meter Run					
81 For Time of: •500-Meter Run •25 Dumbbell Clean and Presses •500-Meter Run •25 Dumbbell Burpees and Presses •500-Meter Run •25 Dumbbell Thrusters •500-Meter Run					

	WORKOUTS	Day 6 Reps / Time / Weight	Day 7 Reps / Time / Weight	Day 8 Reps / Time / Weight	Day 9 Reps / Time / Weight	Day 10 Reps / Time / Weight
76	•5 Rounds for Time of: •20 Dumbbell Floor Press •20 Dumbbell Sumo Squats •20 Dumbbell Thrusters •20 Push-ups					
77	As many reps as possible in 15 minutes of: •10 Dumbbell Push-up with Row (Alternate arms) •10 Dumbbell Snatches •10 Dumbbell Squats					
78	•50 Dumbbell Strict Presses •50 Dumbbell Pull-Overs •50 Dumbbell Bent Over Rows					
79	•50 Dumbbell Man-Makers •1,000-meter Run •25 Dumbbell Devil Presses					
80	For Time of: •1,000-meter Run Then, 3 Rounds for Time of: •8 Dumbbell Burpees to Presses •100-meter Farmer's Carry •8 Dual Dumbbell Overhead Reverse Lunge (Alternate legs) •100 Air Squats Finally, perform: •1,000-meter Run					
81	For Time of: •500-Meter Run •25 Dumbbell Clean and Presses •500-Meter Run •25 Dumbbell Burpees and Presses •500-Meter Run •25 Dumbbell Thrusters •500-Meter Run					

	Day 1	Day 2	Day 3	Day 4	Day 5
WORKOUTS	Reps / Time / Weight	Reps / Time / Weight	Reps / Time / Weight	Reps / Time / Weight	Reps / Time / Weight
82 5 Rounds for Time of: •5 Dumbbell Man-Makers •10 Dumbbell Lunges (Alternate legs) •15 Burpees •20 Push-ups					
83 •500-Meter Run •25 Dumbbell Deadlifts •25 Burpees Over Dumbbells •1,000-Meter Run •25 Dumbbell Deadlifts •25 Burpees Over Dumbbells •500-Meter Run					
84 5 Rounds for Time of: •10 Dumbbell Hang Snatches (Alternate arms) •15 Dumbbell Lunges (Alternate legs) •20 Sit-Ups •25 Burpees					
85 5 Rounds for Time of: •10 Dumbbell Thrusters •15 Push-ups •20 Burpees •25 Air Squats					
86 3 Rounds for Time of: •1,000-Meter Run •25 Dumbbell Squat Cleans •25 Burpees •25 Push-ups					
87 •12 Rounds for Time of: •10 Dumbbell Hang Squat Cleans •10 Dumbbell Hang Clean-and-Jerks (Alternate arms)					

	WORKOUTS	Day 6 Reps / Time / Weight	Day 7 Reps / Time / Weight	Day 8 Reps / Time / Weight	Day 9 Reps / Time / Weight	Day 10 Reps / Time / Weight
82	5 Rounds for Time of: •5 Dumbbell Man-Makers •10 Dumbbell Lunges (Alternate legs) •15 Burpees •20 Push-ups					
83	•500-Meter Run •25 Dumbbell Deadlifts •25 Burpees Over Dumbbells •1,000-Meter Run •25 Dumbbell Deadlifts •25 Burpees Over Dumbbells •500-Meter Run					
84	5 Rounds for Time of: •10 Dumbbell Hang Snatches (Alternate arms) •15 Dumbbell Lunges (Alternate legs) •20 Sit-Ups •25 Burpees					
85	5 Rounds for Time of: •10 Dumbbell Thrusters •15 Push-ups •20 Burpees •25 Air Squats					
86	3 Rounds for Time of: •1,000-Meter Run •25 Dumbbell Squat Cleans •25 Burpees •25 Push-ups					
87	•12 Rounds for Time of: •10 Dumbbell Hang Squat Cleans •10 Dumbbell Hang Clean-and-Jerks (Alternate arms)					

	WORKOUTS	Day 1 Reps / Time / Weight	Day 2 Reps / Time / Weight	Day 3 Reps / Time / Weight	Day 4 Reps / Time / Weight	Day 5 Reps / Time / Weight
88	•12 Rounds for Time of: •250-meter Runs •12 Dumbbell Burpee Deadlifts					
89	For time of 10-9-8-7-6-5-4-3-2-1 Reps of: •Dumbbell Snatches (Alternate arms) •Push-Ups					
90	•5 Rounds for Time of: •15 Dumbbell Deadlifts •30 Sit-ups •15 Dumbbell Shoulder Presses •15 Dumbbell Squat Cleans					
91	2 Rounds for Time of: •20 Dumbbell Goblet Squats •10 Burpees •500-meter Run 2 Rounds for Time of: •20 Dumbbell Walking Lunges •10 v-ups •500-meter Run 2 Rounds for Time of: •20 Dumbbell Squats •1 minute plank hold •500-meter Run 2 Rounds for Time of: •20 Dumbbell Romanian Deadlifts •20 Push-ups •500-meter Run					

		Day 6	Day 7	Day 8	Day 9	Day 10
	WORKOUTS	Reps / Time / Weight	Reps / Time / Weight	Reps / Time / Weight	Reps / Time / Weight	Reps / Time / Weight
88	•12 Rounds for Time of: •250-meter Runs •12 Dumbbell Burpee Deadlifts					
89	For time of 10-9-8-7-6-5-4-3-2-1 Reps of: •Dumbbell Snatches (Alternate arms) •Push-Ups					
90	•5 Rounds for Time of: •15 Dumbbell Deadlifts •30 Sit-ups •15 Dumbbell Shoulder Presses •15 Dumbbell Squat Cleans					
91	2 Rounds for Time of: •20 Dumbbell Goblet Squats •10 Burpees •500-meter Run 2 Rounds for Time of: •20 Dumbbell Walking Lunges •10 v-ups •500-meter Run 2 Rounds for Time of: •20 Dumbbell Squats •1 minute plank hold •500-meter Run 2 Rounds for Time of: •20 Dumbbell Romanian Deadlifts •20 Push-ups •500-meter Run					

	WORKOUTS	Day 1	Day 2	Day 3	Day 4	Day 5
		Reps / Time / Weight	Reps / Time / Weight	Reps / Time / Weight	Reps / Time / Weight	Reps / Time / Weight
92	•100 Russian Twists with Dumbbell •90 Dumbbell Goblet Squats •80 Dumbbell Push Presses •70 Dumbbell Reverse Lunges •60 Dumbbell Snatches (Alternate arms) •50 Dumbbell Power Cleans •40 Dumbbell Overhead Squats (Split reps between arms) •30 Dumbbell Deadlifts					
93	•1000-meter run •50 Dumbbell Snatches (Alternate arms) •50 Sit-Ups •750-meter run •40 Dumbbell Snatches (Alternate arms) •40 Sit-Ups •500-meter run •30 Dumbbell Snatches (Alternate arms) •30 Sit-Ups					
94	5 Rounds for Time of: •15 Dumbbell Thrusters •50 Dumbbell Overhead Reverse Lunge (Alternate legs)					
95	•20 Dumbbell Thrusters •500-meter Run •20 Dumbbell Thrusters •500-meter Run •20 Dumbbell Thrusters •500-meter Run					

	WORKOUTS	Day 6 Reps / Time / Weight	Day 7 Reps / Time / Weight	Day 8 Reps / Time / Weight	Day 9 Reps / Time / Weight	Day 10 Reps / Time / Weight
92	•100 Russian Twists with Dumbbell •90 Dumbbell Goblet Squats •80 Dumbbell Push Presses •70 Dumbbell Reverse Lunges •60 Dumbbell Snatches (Alternate arms) •50 Dumbbell Power Cleans •40 Dumbbell Overhead Squats (Split reps between arms) •30 Dumbbell Deadlifts					
93	•1000-meter run •50 Dumbbell Snatches (Alternate arms) •50 Sit-Ups •750-meter run •40 Dumbbell Snatches (Alternate arms) •40 Sit-Ups •500-meter run •30 Dumbbell Snatches (Alternate arms) •30 Sit-Ups					
94	5 Rounds for Time of: •15 Dumbbell Thrusters •50 Dumbbell Overhead Reverse Lunge (Alternate legs)					
95	•20 Dumbbell Thrusters •500-meter Run •20 Dumbbell Thrusters •500-meter Run •20 Dumbbell Thrusters •500-meter Run					

	WORKOUTS	Day 1 Reps / Time / Weight	Day 2 Reps / Time / Weight	Day 3 Reps / Time / Weight	Day 4 Reps / Time / Weight	Day 5 Reps / Time / Weight
96	3 Rounds for Time of: •11 Dumbbell Snatches (Right arm) •11 Dumbbell Overhead Lunges (Right arm) •11 Dumbbell Snatches (Left arm) •11 Dumbbell Overhead Lunges (Left arm) •11 Dumbbell Power Cleans •11 Dumbbell Front Squats •11 Dumbbell Power Cleans •11 Dumbbell Front Squats					
97	4 Rounds for Time of: •10 Dumbbell Thrusters •20 Burpees •40 Air Squats					
98	3 Rounds for Time of: •1,000-meter Run •30 Burpees •30 Dumbbell Squat Cleans					
99	Part 1: Every minute on the minute for 3 minutes of: •10 Dumbbell Rows (Alternate arms) •10 Push-Ups Part 2: Every minute on the minute for 3 minutes of: •10 Dumbbell Thrusters •10 Push-Ups Part 3: Every minute on the minute for 3 minutes of: •10 Dumbbell Rows (Alternate arms) •10 Push-Ups Part 4: As many rounds as possible in 3 minutes of: •Dumbbell Thrusters					

	WORKOUTS	Day 6 Reps / Time / Weight	Day 7 Reps / Time / Weight	Day 8 Reps / Time / Weight	Day 9 Reps / Time / Weight	Day 10 Reps / Time / Weight
96	3 Rounds for Time of: •11 Dumbbell Snatches (Right arm) •11 Dumbbell Overhead Lunges (Right arm) •11 Dumbbell Snatches (Left arm) •11 Dumbbell Overhead Lunges (Left arm) •11 Dumbbell Power Cleans •11 Dumbbell Front Squats •11 Dumbbell Power Cleans •11 Dumbbell Front Squats					
97	4 Rounds for Time of: •10 Dumbbell Thrusters •20 Burpees •40 Air Squats					
98	3 Rounds for Time of: •1,000-meter Run •30 Burpees •30 Dumbbell Squat Cleans					
99	Part 1: Every minute on the minute for 3 minutes of: •10 Dumbbell Rows (Alternate arms) •10 Push-Ups Part 2: Every minute on the minute for 3 minutes of: •10 Dumbbell Thrusters •10 Push-Ups Part 3: Every minute on the minute for 3 minutes of: •10 Dumbbell Rows (Alternate arms) •10 Push-Ups Part 4: As many rounds as possible in 3 minutes of: •Dumbbell Thrusters					

	WORKOUTS	Day 1 Reps / Time / Weight	Day 2 Reps / Time / Weight	Day 3 Reps / Time / Weight	Day 4 Reps / Time / Weight	Day 5 Reps / Time / Weight
100	21-15-9 Reps for Time of: •Dumbbell Thrusters •Air Squats •Burpees					
101	As many rounds as possible in 20 minutes of: •20 Air Squats •10 Dumbbell Rows (Right arm) •20 Mountain climbers •10 Dumbbell Rows (Left arm) •20 Sit-ups					
102	•5 Rounds of: •10 Dumbbell Thrusters •20 Burpees •30 Plank Shoulder Taps					
103	Every minute on the minute for 15 minutes of: • 10 Dumbbell Snatches (Alternate arms) After each 3 minutes perform •50 Jumping Jacks					
104	10 Rounds for Time of: •200-meter Run •10 Dumbbell Burpee Deadlifts					
105	12 Rounds for Time of: •12 Dumbbell Hang Squat Cleans •12 Push-Ups					
106	5 Rounds for Time of: •15 Dumbbell Man-Makers •25 Dumbbell Deadlifts •35 Dumbbell Snatches (Split reps between arms) •45 Overhead Lunges (Split reps between arms) •55 Dumbbell Swings					

	WORKOUTS	Day 6 Reps / Time / Weight	Day 7 Reps / Time / Weight	Day 8 Reps / Time / Weight	Day 9 Reps / Time / Weight	Day 10 Reps / Time / Weight
100	21-15-9 Reps for Time of: •Dumbbell Thrusters •Air Squats •Burpees					
101	As many rounds as possible in 20 minutes of: •20 Air Squats •10 Dumbbell Rows (Right arm) •20 Mountain climbers •10 Dumbbell Rows (Left arm) •20 Sit-ups					
102	•5 Rounds of: •10 Dumbbell Thrusters •20 Burpees •30 Plank Shoulder Taps					
103	Every minute on the minute for 15 minutes of: • 10 Dumbbell Snatches (Alternate arms) After each 3 minutes perform •50 Jumping Jacks					
104	10 Rounds for Time of: •200-meter Run •10 Dumbbell Burpee Deadlifts					
105	12 Rounds for Time of: •12 Dumbbell Hang Squat Cleans •12 Push-Ups					
106	5 Rounds for Time of: •15 Dumbbell Man-Makers •25 Dumbbell Deadlifts •35 Dumbbell Snatches (Split reps between arms) •45 Overhead Lunges (Split reps between arms) •55 Dumbbell Swings					

	WORKOUTS	Day 1 Reps / Time / Weight	Day 2 Reps / Time / Weight	Day 3 Reps / Time / Weight	Day 4 Reps / Time / Weight	Day 5 Reps / Time / Weight
107	21-15-9 Reps for Time of: •Dumbbell Thrusters •Air Squats •Push-ups •Burpees					
108	•12 Dumbbell Bent Over Rows •12 Dumbbell Ground-to-Overheads (Split reps between arms) •10 Up-Downs + Mountain Climbers •10 Dumbbell Bent Over Rows •10 Dumbbell Ground-to-Overheads •10 Up-Downs + Mountain Climbers •8 Dumbbell Bent Over Rows •8 Dumbbell Ground-to-Overheads •10 Up-Downs + Mountain Climbers					
109	4 Rounds for Time of: •20 Dumbbell Thrusters •500-meter Run •20 Burpees					
110	For Time: •20 Dumbbell Devil Presses •50 Dumbbell Thrusters •80 Burpees					
111	As many rounds as possible in 20 minutes of: •5 Dumbbell Thrusters •5 Push-ups •5 Dumbbell Deadlifts •5 Dumbbell Devil Presses					

WORKOUTS		Day 6 Reps / Time / Weight	Day 7 Reps / Time / Weight	Day 8 Reps / Time / Weight	Day 9 Reps / Time / Weight	Day 10 Reps / Time / Weight
107	21-15-9 Reps for Time of: •Dumbbell Thrusters •Air Squats •Push-ups •Burpees					
108	•12 Dumbbell Bent Over Rows •12 Dumbbell Ground-to-Overheads (Split reps between arms) •10 Up-Downs + Mountain Climbers •10 Dumbbell Bent Over Rows •10 Dumbbell Ground-to-Overheads •10 Up-Downs + Mountain Climbers •8 Dumbbell Bent Over Rows •8 Dumbbell Ground-to-Overheads •10 Up-Downs + Mountain Climbers					
109	4 Rounds for Time of: •20 Dumbbell Thrusters •500-meter Run •20 Burpees					
110	For Time: •20 Dumbbell Devil Presses •50 Dumbbell Thrusters •80 Burpees					
111	As many rounds as possible in 20 minutes of: •5 Dumbbell Thrusters •5 Push-ups •5 Dumbbell Deadlifts •5 Dumbbell Devil Presses					

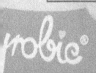

BONUS No 1 - ALL LOGGING SHEETS of this book are available through this QR code that you can use to scan, print, and record your workouts to measure your performance as many times you want

Dear valued customer,

We are a small family-owned business, and we'd like to please kindly ask you to leave us a review.

We don't have the same budget as big publishing companies, so your support would be really appreciated. Your feedback will mean a lot to us, and we thank you in advance!

Mauricio & Devon

BONUS No 2 - VIDEOS for ALL EXERCISES ARE AVAILABLE HERE. If you want check how the exercises are to be performed, scan the QR codes with your mobile device.

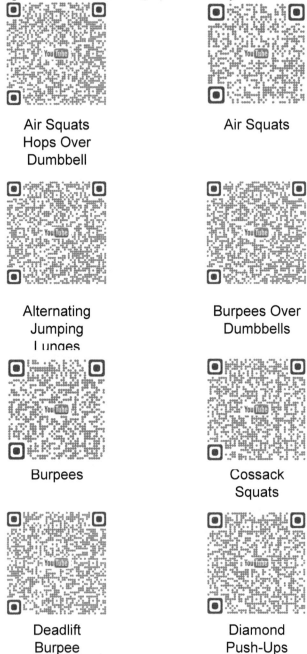

Air Squats Hops Over Dumbbell

Air Squats

Alternating Jumping Lunges

Burpees Over Dumbbells

Burpees

Cossack Squats

Deadlift Burpee Dumbbells

Diamond Push-Ups

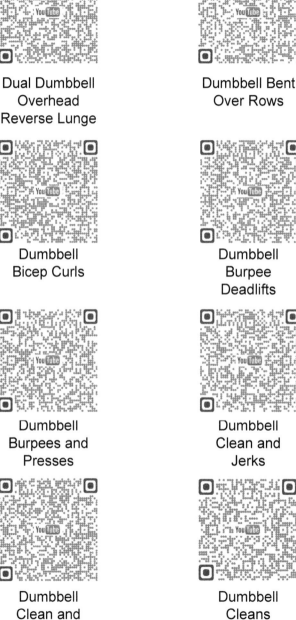

Dual Dumbbell Overhead Reverse Lunge	Dumbbell Bent Over Rows
Dumbbell Bicep Curls	Dumbbell Burpee Deadlifts
Dumbbell Burpees and Presses	Dumbbell Clean and Jerks
Dumbbell Clean and Presses	Dumbbell Cleans

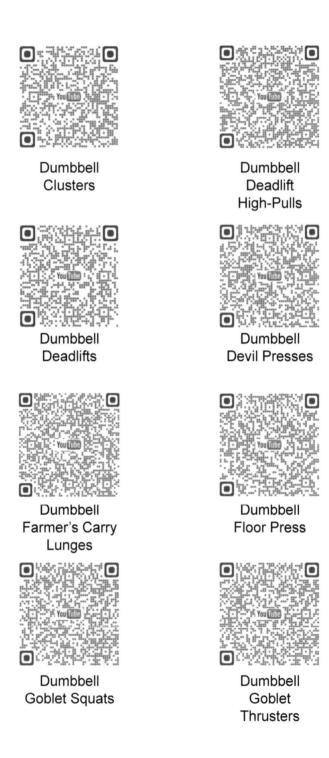

Dumbbell
Ground-to-Over
head

Dumbbell
Hammer Curls

Dumbbell
Hammer Curls

Dumbbell
Hand Power
Cleans

Dumbbell
Hang Clean
Thrusters

Dumbbell Hang
Clean-and-Jerks

Dumbbell
Hang Cleans

Dumbbell
Hang
High-Pulls

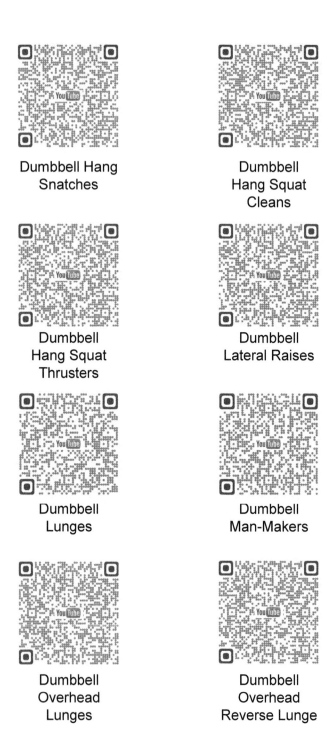

Dumbbell Hang Snatches

Dumbbell Hang Squat Cleans

Dumbbell Hang Squat Thrusters

Dumbbell Lateral Raises

Dumbbell Lunges

Dumbbell Man-Makers

Dumbbell Overhead Lunges

Dumbbell Overhead Reverse Lunge

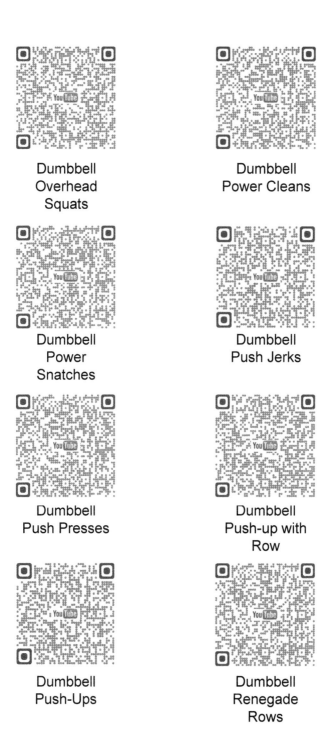

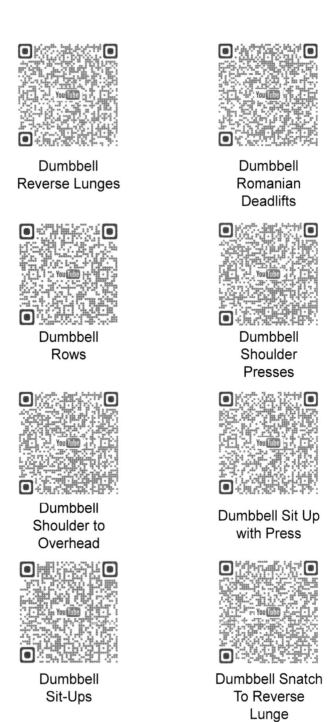

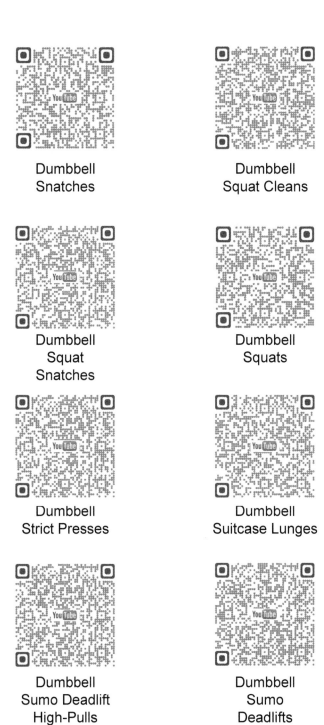

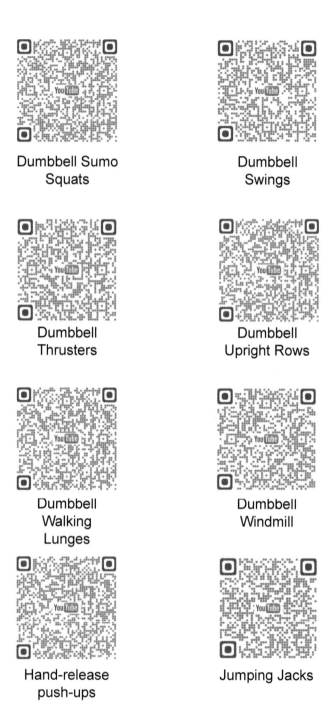

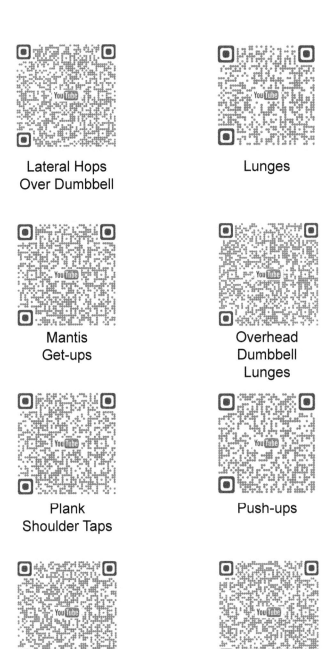

Single-Arm
Dumbbell Strict
Presses

Sit-Ups

Spider-Man
Push-Ups

Up-Downs +
Mountain
Climbers

V-Ups

www.ingramcontent.com/pod-product-compliance
Lightning Source LLC
LaVergne TN
LVHW022337200625
814209LV00008B/389